Raising Twins - A Journey:

Modern Techniques to Being the Best Parent you Can Be.

by Casey Florence

In case you just realized you are going to have twins for the first time or second time, all you need to do is to calm yourself down because you are going to pull through. But be sure you and your manifold will have a whole new experience. First thing you need to pay attention to is your health because you have to take care of yourself and stay healthy so you can be strong enough to cater for this double blessing.

Secondly, knowing what to expect and how to handles it is very important. However, you need not to worry if you don't know what to expect because you are not alone. Not having an idea of what to expect is common amongst most women expecting twins but it doesn't stop them from learning these things. Believe me, it is an interesting and promising experience that will definitely oust the fears as the new lifestyle sync in.

Another thing most expecting mothers worry about is how they survive.

This book will give you great insight and help you stay optimistic as well as ensuring that your expectation matches up with your preparations. This will prevent you from having long and stressful early months filled with tiring activities like feeding, changing nappies and of course sleepless nights.

Thanks you for taking interest in my book and I hope you have an amazing double blessed journey!

Contents

Chapter 1

Staying healthy and lowering complications while pregnant

There are mothers who are "high risk" when carrying twins or more than one child, but not all are. This should not therefore intimidate you because it may mean that you will only need to be monitored closely, but not that you will have problems. However, there are mothers who experience various complications while pregnant. Some have diabetes, which may magnify in pregnancy, while some have previous preterm labor, which leads to premature birth in prior pregnancies, and others have pre-existing health conditions.

Some of the complications arising from the pregnancy and delivery of twins include:

Morning sickness

Morning sickness may be worse with twin pregnancies. Although it is called morning sickness, it can happen any time with or without vomiting, but it is usually worse in the morning. Nausea and vomiting, especially first thing in the morning is also common in some pregnant women. Usually these symptoms of morning sickness disappear by the second trimester.

Preeclampsia

Preeclampsia is Pregnancy Induced Hypertension. PIH is more common with twin pregnancies and it can be either mild or severe. It will be detected when high blood pressure is measured or when there is excess protein in the urine. You should consult your health care professional if you notice swelling on your face, hands or feet so it can be treated early. If preeclampsia is not treated there could be higher risks of preterm labor or premature birth.

Premature labor

When labor occurs before 37 weeks, it is known as premature labor. Many mothers experience labor between 36-38 weeks for multiple births. The fact that you are expecting twins does not mean that you will not carry the pregnancy to term and have a natural birth, because many mothers have done so. Discuss with your doctor any signs and prevention measures of preterm labor. If you are able to recognize signs of premature labor early, it can easily be prevented.

Prevention of premature labor includes:

- Get enough sleep and rest, put your feet up in bed or on the couch if it is possible, take naps during the day. Sleep on your side, especially the left side to relieve the pressure on your uterus and increase blood flow.

- Attend a prenatal clinic to have your <u>pregnancy</u> monitored by your doctor.

- Always listen to your body language and call your doctor if you notice anything odd. Early detection is the best solution for successful treatment of preterm labor. Once premature labor has been diagnosed, you will be given medications to stop or slow down labor, antibiotics for any infections and complete or partial bed rest may help. In the worst instances, you may be admitted to hospital for treatment for induced labor or C-section.

Preterm birth

When babies are born before 37 weeks it is known as preterm birth, but with proper they will grow just as fine as any other babies. Report any concerns you may have to your doctor. The doctor may induce labor or perform a C-section if there are complications, so that both you and your babies are safe.

Cesarean section

Cesarean section deliveries may be more common with twin pregnancies than for singletons. There are many deliveries done through C-section, especially multiple births. This depends on how the babies are lying in the womb and if there are any complications. Both children can be delivered this way, or one child may have been born normally and the second child through C-section if complications arise. However, you should know that people are different and every birth is unique.

The C-section may be performed when:-

- the pelvis is too small or the baby's head is too big
- the babies are breech; lying sideways
- the mother has a hemorrhage due to uterine rupture making her lose a lot of blood
- the fetuses are in distress due to lack of oxygen or poor blood flow
- labor is not progressing the way it should if the cervix has not opened up
- there is placenta praevia or placenta abruption
- there is a cord prolapse which limits supply of oxygen

- the mother had prior caesarean births although she can also deliver naturally

- preeclampsia is causing low blood flow and oxygen supply

You must attend all prenatal appointments so that the doctor can detect any problems early. Discuss any complications with the doctor like swelling, spotting and pain so you can get advice and preventive treatment.

Chapter 2

Going Home: The Early Days and Weeks

So how do you make it through this tough transitional period? It is important for you and your partner to have your own space and alone time at least once a day or twice every month as you start on this journey, and then make more time for each other as your twins age and have fewer dependencies.

The Early Months: Giving your twins the best upbringing

Women excitedly imagine dressing up their two little ones in matching clothes, taking pictures of them, and loads of fun on play time, what they often forget is all the effort, time, energy, money and lifestyle changes that comes with welcoming twins into their life. The stress can really take its toll on parents and you'll possibly find yourself screaming out frustrations at your partner since you can't at your baby, as your resort to release stress. It's all okay though, depending on how understanding your partner is. Unfortunately, for this reason and more, marital relationships often take the hit when twins are born. Don't fear though, having twins has its own blessings and wonders, it is just a reality that having twins can put a huge tension on a relationship, especially if you are un-prepared on this journey to parenthood.

Another reason many marriages experience a huge amount of stress in the first year of having twins. Is baby twins demand a lot of energy and time. So keeping your multiples on the same schedule is very important. Growing into a routine-oriented parenting habit is advisable for you to cope more easily. Setting a staggered schedule to take care of your twins, making sure ach has your undivided attention for feeding, playtime, and prepping for naptime. And being able to have as much rest as humanly possible every day, is critical for you to be able to cope with these demands.

Adjusting to New Patterns

Every baby is different and has their own sleep patterns. To cope through the night and your schedule, it's ideal to have babies in bed at the same time every night. If one baby wakes up, wake up his/her twin too (and yes, it's one of the rare times it's okay to disrupt a baby's sleep). This will soon set their body clocks on the same times for changing, feeding, sleeping on schedule.

Form and follow through a bedtime routine. Babies develop habits through consistency, so develop a bedtime routine that fits you and your babies best. Bath, books or music, than bed seems to be the standard flowchart routine that works best. Make this time fun and stress-free, and it will make for great bonding time between you and your twins.

Lay them to bed drowsy, but still awake. You don't want them to develop sleep crutches (not being able to fall asleep) especially considering you have twins. It may seem sweet and harmless to rock or feed your babies to sleep, but if they get too used to it, they'll need you every time they wake up, including in the middle of the night. The goal of this is to train them to get act on their sleepiness and sleep on their own.

Coping with Broken Sleep Patterns.

Lets face ot everyone gets cranky without enough sleep and it will be unavoidable the first few months with your multiples. But there are ways for you to cope with. Take quick 15 minute power naps when you start feeling tired during the day. They're not long but they will make a huge difference with your coping and energy, and will also keep you from falling asleep accidentally. Just keep your babies in a secure place and catch some shut eye, and make sure to set an alarm so you don't oversleep.

Remember with raising multiples, you and your partner are both at work, so the burden of broken sleep in the nights should be shared as much as possible. If needed find a way for both of you to get a break and recover some time by asking a relative to help or even a 'night nanny' who is available to work a night-time shift for caring while you and your spouse catch up on much needed sleep.

If your twins start bottle-feeding, you can opt to take turns as partners to handle the night care alternately. Some couples agree on shifts for the first few weeks or months, since these times demand more wake times at night with more feedings and diaper changes. For example, one parent can nap and cover caring for the twins from 7pm till 1am while the other sleeps; then the other swaps to take the next shift from 1am to 7am while the other takes his/her turn to sleep. This way both parents are guaranteed at least a fixed amount of sleep and a chance to recover.

Co-Cribbing

While they are still small, you can opt to have your twins sleep in a single crib, either because there's not much space or that they slept in one together when they were in the hospital. It's called co-cribbing, and it's perfectly safe. Actually, keeping twins in one crib can help them keep their body temperatures regulated and help with their sleep cycles, while also soothing both of them. You can opt to keep co-cribbing until they reach about six months or until they start to roll over.

If you do decide to put your twins in one crib, place them on their backs with the tops of their heads, in a face to face position with each other while their feet are at opposite ends of the crib, or side by side back-to-back, with their feet positioned at the foot of the crib.

It's also best to consult with a pediatrician if you plan on co-cribbing your twins.

Generally, here's what you need to consider:

The Set Up

You can opt for a "twin crib" that has a division in the center that can hold both babies. A lot of your choices and decisions will be based on the behavior and adjustment of your twins in a co-sleeping set-up. Some get along with it very well, but few babies end up waking the other twin. It is best to have some flexibility as you figure out what works best for your babies.

As your twins get older, you can opt to have them in two separate cribs placed close to each other, so they can still comfort each other as they sleep. For the 1st six months, it's also suggested parents have their babies sleep in the same room as theirs. However, if you find that one baby disturbs the other, you might want to provide them separate rooms at an older age (If you have the space).

More tips:

- Using a Moses basket to co-crib is not advisable, it has very limited space and poses a risk of overheating.
- Avoid cross-contamination of illness between twins if one baby is sick
- Co-cribbing is also not advisable if one of the twins has a birth defect, e.g. downs, spina bifida, it would be safer for the babies to be in separate cribs
- A baby's sleep is important for their health, so keep tab of sleep disturbances, and stability of temperature when deciding if the setup works or not
- Babies with a low birth weight (below 2.5kg or 5.5lbs) or that were born premature, younger than 37 weeks (multiples often fall in this group) are at risk of crib death, so it very important that all the advice on reducing the risk of crib death is followed
- Due to the higher risk of crib death, when you decide to co-crib triplets and higher multiples, it is very important for parents to keep a very close eye on them, it is best to move them around and becoming more mobile, following as much advice a on reducing the risk of crib death is very important in this case.

Chapter 3

Using your budget wisely for your twins

Setting up and decorating a the layette and nursery for twins, can be both fun and frustrating. So when you're shopping for the nursery, think for the long term, you'll want to buy quality fixtures and furniture that can grow with your kids.

Don't go for a secondhand car seat. There are expiration dates for car seats, they also aren't supposed to be used after a car accident. You will find the expiration date printed on the bottom of the car seat. Usually, the expiration is 3-5 years after its manufacturing.

You also won't always be able to tell if the car seat has been in an accident if you buy secondhand. Safety1st.com is a recommended store when buying car seats. They have very affordable car seats with a wide range to choose from. It can seem fun to put in extra fixtures to your baby's car seat like a head bumper, or other accessories, but these "after market" items void the car seat's warranty. So it is best to only use the things that came with the car seat when you bought it.

A changing table is not a necessity. Changing your twin's clothes and diapers on the floor, the bed, and the couch and other places offer the same convenience as a changing table. A changing table doesn't really offer any additional advantage. If you are certain you really want a setup like that, you can find dressers that have a built-in changing pad on top.

As a smart a mom you will want to buy stuff that has multiple uses. Items tend to be obsolete sooner if they have only one use. Like instead of a diaper pail, just buy a plastic bin or trash can that closes all the way. They when you're done using for dirty diapers you can clean it and reuse it for other things like a trash can or toy basket. The goal is to buy things you can use later for other things.

Try to avoid being impulsive when buying "things", especially for the first 2-4 weeks, your attention and time will be focused more on feeding, sleeping, changing diapers, and calming down the crying. There won't be much use for toys yet during this time. You'll be surprised how much laundry your little ones produce in a single day, from bibs, blankets and clothes.

Assign some little zones in your home for you and your babies. Include a feeding zone with snacks and activities for you, a napping or resting zone where you can steal some time to rest but have them in hearing range, a neutral activity zone where you complete some chores or tasks while still spending time with your twins.

What You Will Absolutely Need

Buy classic furniture and fixture that can last and transform as your children get older. Consider cribs that you can later convert to toddler beds and then can later be used. A changing table will be quite a waste as once your twins are potty trained or grow too big for it you won't have any use for it. You can instead opt to buy an inexpensive yet plush changing pad and set it up on top of your babies' dresser to save some money.

Stick to cheap but smart stuff. Don't get tempted by the stuff labelled as a "need" in Babies R Us. More than all that, your children are going to need breast milk, safety, comfort, warmth, and clean diapers.

Laying down the Clothing Layette.

If your situation calls for doing laundry regularly, and you are not getting hand me downs,, here's a basic layette list of everything you should buy for your twins.

10 to 12 soft onesies
10 to 12 one piece, pajamas
3 to 4 soft fabric sweaters
2 to 3 sets of baby boots
6 to 10 blankies
2-dozen diapers of any variation
10 to 12 bibs
3 to 4 crib sheets (for each crib)

2 crib mattresses (for each crib)
2 sheets to cover the changing pad
10 to 12 socks
3 to 4 warm hats

Items to Skip:

Crib bedding / bumpers

Baby Thermometers.

Special baby thermometers aren't a necessity, it's just marketing creating a need. Even Pediatricians use and say the regular digital thermometers (the same ones you use as an adult) will work just as fine for babies.

The diaper bag.

A bag specific just for baby's diapers isn't a necessity. That and any bag just for wipes or other necessities on-the-go can be easily organized in one regular backpack. It's another thing you can be smart about on your budget.

A hands-free pumping bra.

This is an instant $40 savings if you can get creative with an old sports bra. You can just cut two holes in it, and there you have it! A DIY hands-free pumping bra.

Bottle Warmer

You can use a basin or a large cup fill it with water and place the bottles there for a few minutes

Mobiles

Baby gloves

Baby socks will do just as fine if you want to keep your baby from scratching themselves

Glider

For one, it isn't big enough to hold twins. You can opt for a full sized recliner, you can even snuggle in with the twins while reading stories.

Don't feel embarrassed to ask for help, your family and friends have growing children are probably excited to give old stuff away.

Chapter 4

Twins: Two Distinct Individuals

Even with identical twins, no twins will ever be exactly alike. Each baby will have their own unique personality and disposition. They will have their own particular intellectual weaknesses and strengths. Even when they're like two peas in a pod, you will find that they will interact and develop with their environment differently from one another.

As twins grow older, their sense of individuality is often encouraged by parents. Now that doesn't necessarily mean that you cannot celebrate their unique special twin bond, but having their identity as an individual is also important for each of them to develop well, not just seeing themselves as "one of a pair".

Calling the babies "the boys", "the girls" or "the twins," is a common trap Parents, family members, and friends fall into. While this may seem harmless, it can affect the twin's sense of individuality and can make them feel under-appreciated as individuals. It is ideal to try to call them by their own names separately, instead of referring to them as a "borg". You should also try to change the order of their names when you call or address them: for example, instead of always calling "Lea and Lila," change it up a sometimes and call them Lila and Lea. This will keep any one of the twins from feeling like they're second best. Another thing to avoid is using labels. Keep from labelling any of duo as "the athletic one" "the smart one" "the adventurous one" etc. this limits their self-esteem, affecting their development and potential.

Self-Reliance

While teaching your children about teamwork in the family, teaching them about self-reliance is equally as valuable. A child's ability to depend on themselves, allows them to develop their own strengths and understand how to use it to achieve specific goals. If they constantly relying on the family or each other for help, it keeps them from learning to become independent. And though this may not always be a bad thing as seeing our children working together instead of wrangling at each other is always a better prospect. Children will also encounter challenges and situations when they are alone and will need to be able to handle that themselves. Teaching children about self-reliance could include tasks or specific chores that are meant for only one of them to complete.

Don't forget that each of the twins are individual persons, so keep this in mind even as you teach them about working together. If they both like dressing alike and they share the same preferences for other things, then that's perfectly fine. Just remember that our individual choices is one of the things that makes humans unique and special, it is how we develop as individuals and should be embraced with wide open arms.

Chapter 5

Outing advice and essentials to have when leaving home.

Going out for an adventure outdoors? You'll find that travelling with your twins will be an adventure on its own. From getting ready for the trip to going out and being out with them.

You'll have to consider a lot the logistics when caring for multiples. One baby alone is already unpredictable on a trip, anything can go wrong. The possibility of that becomes higher when you have multiples. You'll have to take care of two little ones who each have their own specific comfort levels and their appetite for feeding. Then you have changing diapers, or clothes and any other needs... Couples tend to go anti-social as even simply going out on a date can be quite a challenge.

Well, let me tell you with resounding clear confidence—you can make it happen!

Start by easing into it. Don't get all too excited and make plans for whole day of activities every Saturday. Start by activities that take a couple of hours. It is more realistic to manage and make for time that less likely causes a meltdown. Overstimulated babies will get you and your babies stressed. Try on winning over the easier challenges like going out for a quick trip to the grocery or farmer's market. Save the bigger ones for when you and your babies are ready, for now avoid a whole day at the beach or an all-day shopping at the mall. Easing into it allows you the chance to develop a system that works while understanding your babies' temperament outside the house and in the car.

When you're going out shopping with your little ones, speed is the key to success. Have a plan in mind before you go so you can get the stuff, and get out. This could mean that you won't have the luxury of comparing products or trying things on. But reviews are available online, you can plan ahead on what to check so you can make the most of your time. You can decide then what looks right, and remember that it all doesn't have to be in one trip. You can return what doesn't fit or doesn't work out with another trip.

It also helps a lot to know which stores have the most restrooms, and to know where they are. Then check which ones have changing tables, and the best ones are the ones that have family rooms where you have more space to take care of, feed and change your twin babies.

You'll find that the multitude of strangers who feel compelled to greet and touch your babies and chat with you, is one of the biggest interference when taking your twins out for a trip to the grocery store or when running an errand. Seeing your twins seems to send them off into a spree of stories about every person in their life who has twins (like you care, right?), and then there's the inevitable cliché question of "How could you ever tell them apart?" And that's even if your twins are totally fraternal, they will still seem identical to strangers. There are a few tips you can follow but they go against some manners and might be out of the comfort zone on your side. But hey, no one said it was not going to be a transition, right lol?

Firstly, avoid eye contact even from those obviously trying to talk to you. You can easily tell whom your twins have caught whose attention by listening. You will hear comments like "aww" or "double trouble" or "oh, look" or "wow, she sure has her hands full," just keep your head down or straight and carry on. Otherwise, you will have to deal with every one of them and you'll never get your shopping done. Don't attract unwarranted attention by dressing them up alike or encouraging an exhibition of cuteness.

Because you'll find that total strangers are completely comfortable touching and talking to your twins. Some babies might even enjoy the attention, and some babies get stressed over it, so depending on your babies personalities, this can make your trip harder or easier.

The simple trick is if you want to avoid being bothered by strangers, or not have the time to entertain them, you will have to be a bit of a snob and just have to keep moving.

As you start going out with your twins all by yourself, it may feel troublesome and tedious, but going out, having fun, and enjoying it is important. Family adventures make for fond memories and are a lot of fun. They don't have to be extravagant either. It can be a picnic at your favorite park or just a short day out for breakfast or lunch. You will appreciate the experience, feel fulfilled and proud that you did it, and also have more confidence and feel more comfortable to plan and have your next family adventure.

Essentials to Have When Leaving Home.

For both twins, you have to make sure you have all these when your outing:

- Enough Diapers for the trip
- Baby wipes.
- Part of your changing kit for when you have to change poopy bottoms and clean up a mess.
- Bottles and Milk

You can opt to bring your own cool full sized bottles packed with their pair of clean nipples. Car bottle warmers are also available and can be helpful on a trip.

- Extra Burp clothes

In case there are accidents that get you dirty (vomit, spilled juice or milk)

- New changes of clothing.

Anything can happen. Anything, so pack a couple.

- Binkies

If your babies are on pacifiers, you don't want to end in a panic buying at the grocery or pharmacy. Keep a pacifier holder, it's just a little box that snaps close, and attach it to your baby bag, and of course always pack a spare! Your babies can throw them and drop them and even lose them, so be ready rather than sorry.

- Double Snap n' Go Stroller

Get the ones that already have matching car seats or are compatible with your baby car seats.

- Head support for the car (a rolled up receiving blanket will do the trick)
- Baby food and snacks

Pack enough for a meal plus extra in case any of it spills, and bring about 2-3 spoons so you have extra if any of it drops and you find no sink near for you to rinse it.

- 2 Bibs (for each baby)
- Washcloths
- Hand sanitizer.

A mom's best friend.

If it's hot, like in Spring or Summer:

- Sunscreen
- A cooler bag with juice
- Sun hats if applicable

If it's Winter:

- Scarfs and Warmers
- Warm Hats
- Mittens

Alternatives to Outings with Twins.

The World Wide Web gives you access to many things, including grocery shopping. A click of the mouse can get you diapers, milk, groceries, and clothing (both for the little ones and yourself). Still, you don't want to go hermit mode and just hide in the house, you should still go out with your twins occasionally. Online access can be your breakaway, but there will still be a lot of occasions for bonding with your little ones, so don't worry and get clicking.

Wonderful Fun at Home

A warm bath is a pleasure any time of the day. You can have some fun with your twins at the tub, and they can enjoy getting all cleaned up too. Of course, you'll still want to supervise their safety in the tub, but you'll love seeing them having so much fun you might even jump in!

The Messy Mixes

Messy is fun! Even experts say that exposing your child with this form of play is good for their brain development. All the ingredients you need for this recipe of fun is just around the house. Innocent messy projects will keep your little ones busy and entertained for hours. Get those little hands into some finger painting, they will love it!

Chapter 6

Seeking Support

Having a good doctor for your baby is something that is very important to any parent (of twins or not). The doctor will be there for your twins from the moment of their birth and as they grow. Regular checkups with their pediatrician will start frequently at younger ages, and become less frequent as your babies grow into kids.

Given how important a pediatrician's support is to your children, how do you pick the right one? You can ask for recommendations from family and friends who also have children, or you can reach out to your family doctor or even the Obstetrician taking care of you during pregnancy. Advice from the local club of Moms of Multiples can also help, As they have experience caring for multiples. You might even find that they may be even better qualified to give advice.

Running Short of Recommendations?

If you ever find that you aren't getting any recommendations, as sometimes even family or friends don't like the pediatricians they've consulted, you can also look for recommendations online. There are sites that provide a list of doctors in your area, like the American Academy of Pediatrics or even Yelp. You'll find that online reviews aren't just for restaurants or venues around town, they also cover doctors and medical facilities.

The important questions you should think about when choosing a pediatrician are:

- Considering your twins' genders, will you want them both to be seen by a female or male doctor, or will you prefer to have you son seen by a male doctor and your daughter seen by a female doctor?
- Is there enough space in their examination rooms for multiple babies or children?
- What is the reputation of this doctor?
- Is your doctor addressing you as parents or does he/she talk to your children as well?
- As the need may arise (like if both of them are sick) or even for regular check-ups, will this doctor be willing to see both of the simultaneously in one appointment?
- Does the pediatrician have other patients who are twins or any experience with twins?

- Is the clinic staff helpful and pleasant?
- Is the clinic's location convenient and accessible to you?
- Are the doctor's services covered by health insurance?

The Bottom Line

Your personal experience and impressions are important when choosing a doctor so don't ignore them. It is also important that your personality is compatible with your doctor's to avoid any conflict. The pediatrician you choose will be sharing involvement in your children's life and growth, so you will want someone you can both trust and respect you as a parent.

Chapter 7

Toddler Safety

You've probably heard of baby proofing, the same applies of course when you're caring for twin toddlers in the house. It is best to have carpeted floors throughout your home. Having a walk-through baby gate at the top of any staircase is a necessity for safety. Don't get too comfortable thinking your babies will stick to their stuffed animals, toy boxes, or other distractions you keep in the house. Your babies will love to explore and go outside to what is unknown. You can be sure they will go looking for trouble as they explore.

Choose the right spot in the room. That means a spot away from anything they can pull or grab and anything they can easily get hurt from. This includes blind cords, curtains and draperies, windows, desk lamps, wall or floor lamps, radiators, and electrical sockets.

You want to avoid the risk of your babies getting trapped between the bed and the wall. So you can either build the rails on both sides or leave enough space on both sides of the bed while making sure the headboard is flat against the wall.

You can place cushions for any falls from the bed like a soft rug, pillows or a sleeping bag.

Also important is that there are no loose joints, screws or other parts of the hardware, so check this regularly.

Got Crib-climbing Toddlers? Get a sleep sack.

When your babies start reaching their mobility milestones (from crawling, standing, to walking on two feet) early. You'll find that they will want to start exploring more and try to escape their crib. Opting for a sleep sack, in this case, could be ideal for your twins. Sleep sacks leave enough space for your babies to move comfortably, while keeping your babies' legs and feet enclosed, this leaves and keeps them from the mobility to climb. Minimal restrictions like this could be enough to keep your twins from doing any climbing in the middle of the night.

Playground Safety for Twin Toddlers

I have two to keep an eye at the playground when there's only one of me? How do I keep them both safe?

Yes, it can seem impossible to chase after both twins, as you could end up chasing after one while the other hands dangerously on the edge of the play house or monkey bar. It's one of the scariest things a mom with twins has to manage. You know you can't definitely keep them together so how do you keep them both safe during play? Choosing the right playground is key.

Nowadays there are a lot of toddler specific playgrounds, and you can also find outdoor playgrounds that are fenced and away from the road. It is also best to schedule playground visits during times when traffic is light. A smaller and less crowded park is an even better choice, as it will allow you to keep a better eye on them.

When you get to your chosen playground, show and direct your twins to the safer play equipment. You can start with sandbox, it's one place that will keep them busy for long, and they'll find it enjoyable too: You can bring lots of toys for them to use. You can also show them the swings and try to get them to take swings side by side — you'll have them both in one place making it easier for you to watch over them.

Safe zones

An alternative to make watching over energetic toddler twins easier. Is making use of the zoning we covered earlier by assigning a "toddler safe zone". It can be quite an advantage and be designated in a spare room or one area of the house.

Now you might be thinking a playpen should be an easy fix, but even with just one baby, you'll find it won't be enough to hold all that energy in, let alone for twins or multiples. So instead of a playpen, you might want to consider a play yard. Ideally, a good play yard is made up of a series of panels. A gate enclosure can be connected to the play yard too. Panels for the play yard can be made of either wood, plastic, or metal. Look for one with higher panels (play yard panel range from 26" to 30" high). Yards with higher panels have a longer life, and it also makes your children less likely to climb out or their play space.

Baby monitors

Another important tool for baby safety is a video baby monitor, especially for when you're busy with chores. Baby monitors are ideal for use whether your twins sleep in the same room or in separate rooms.

A single monitor would prove sufficient enough if your twins sleep in the one room, and close to each other, even if you prefer a monitor with video. Meanwhile, twins who sleep in separate rooms, don't require having to buy 2 separate monitors. A good buy would be a monitor like the Motorola MBP36S, which can be used on 2 different rooms. You can also buy extra cameras that you can connect to its system. It easily syncs up and allows you to view all connected cameras simultaneously in one scream (like your own CCTV system).

Whichever route you consider, monitoring tools are a necessity for ensuring your children's safety.

Chapter 8

Twin Speech Development and Delay

There isn't much information as to why speech delay tends to be higher in twins and multiples, but there are some theories. For example, many twins seem to share a special connection and easily understand each other's gestures and cues, as a result, they have less need to speak about it. To add, most parents of multiples aren't able to devote enough quality individual one-on-one time with their multiples, they often feel too overwhelmed. The tendency for parents is to give short directions and questions like "stop it" or "come here" or "thirsty?" instead of using full sentences like "Lily, please come here to mommy" or "Would like something to drink?"

Don't get tempted to use "baby talk" no matter how cute you think it is. And when you hear your twins speak mispronounced words, repeat it back to them with the correct word while emphasizing the sounds in the words. Now don't expect that they can immediately perfect it, and instead praise them whenever they try so as not to discourage them. Your role is to let them know what is correct, so it registers with them that way. If all you use around you twins is baby talk. That's all they will learn to use, and it may be cute now, but it won't be when their 3 or 4 years old and every other kid their age is speaking better.

So how can you support your children's speech development better?

Speech and/or language delay in twins and multiples are often caused by many factors:

- Twin Talk. Multiples and twins seem to instinctively develop their own code, spoken language, gestures and body language, that are understandable mostly to just them. This type of communication between them tends to be very effective with each other that they lose the need to speak hence, the delay in their speech.
- The rate of speech and language development in children also tends to be influenced by differences in personality and gender. For one, boys tend to be less verbal than girls and communicate more with gestures, and children who are naturally shy or apprehensive tend to be less talkative

- The demands of raising multiples tend to limit the one-on-one time parents are able to give to each individual child.
- There are also situations where one of the twins or multiples develop speech earlier and tend to own the role as communicator, speaking for their twin/siblings. When twins or multiples have an older sibling, this can happen to, in the case when their sibling does the talking for them.

Here are some language milestones to monitor:

Between 12-24 months:

- Use a combination of two simple words
- Be able to use a vocabulary of 10 – 20 words
- Imitate some animal sounds if you like
- Wave their hands good-bye

Notes: A lot of Health Services Programs specific for Speech and Language are also available for free.

• Get your little ones to copy your sounds and actions. You can help by making it fun with action songs like "Pat-A-Cake", "Itsy Bitsy Spider" and "Wheels on the Bus", and other games like, clapping your hands, making rocket ships sounds, blowing kisses or "Peek-A-Boo".

Other things you can do to encourage language development include:

• For at least 30 minutes every day, give your babies the chance to listen to other noises around them by turning off the TV and radio. You can use this to explain the sounds they are hearing like the car, or dogs barking, the birds or even the washing machine.

• Your babies will experiment with different sounds as they try to play with their mouth and vocal skills to learn to speak. Listen and respond to them as they do.

• Use their names with eye contact, and spend time conversing with each of your children individually every day

• Encourage members of the family, older siblings, and friends to have one-on-one conversations with your babies in the same way.

Keep in mind that you are the best person to help your twins develop. And since you have your little ones and yourself, you're a established language group. And you are their best speech coach!

Chapter 9

Diapering for Twins

Assign and Set up your designated changing space specific for nappy changes in the house. Everything you will be using for changing diapers should be within arm's reach, including diaper rash cream, wipes and baby powder. There should never be any reason for you to leave your baby on a changing table just to grab something. Not even for a second! Always fasten the belt and have a good grip of your baby to avoid any falls. And no matter how rowdy or cranky they may both be never ever put both babies in the changing table at the same time! You can only manage to change one of them anyway, so keep one of your twins in a safe place while you change the other.

Choosing the right diapers:

There's definitely no way around doubling amount for diapers when you have twins. Until your babies reach the potty trained stage, you will have to deal with diapers and lots of them!

Like any other parent, you will have to make the decision on what diaper to use, cloth, disposable, what brand?

To start, there's no big difference when choosing between brands. And be it cloth or disposable, your baby will get rashes and feel uncomfortable if you leave them wearing a soiled diaper for long. Though disposable diapers have some benefits, like having moisturizer and being breathable, some babies tend to be allergic or easily irritated by the chemicals that make them absorbent. Some babies seem to prefer the comfort of soft cloth diapers the most.

Prices

Typically, for two years, you'll find yourself spending between $2000 and $3000 on disposable diapers for each baby. If you opt for cloth diapers and accessories, the cost would be around $800 to $1000 if you do the laundry yourself. If you have them washed through a cloth diaper laundering service, the cost comes close to buying disposable diapers ranging from $2500 to $2800. The difference would be that cloth diapers are reusable for other future babies in the family to use.

Convenience

In the past with diapers, you would have to follow through complicated folds and scary pins, nowadays, cloth diapers are made with buttons, snap closures and Velcro, making it just as easy to change babies' dirty diapers as disposable ones. They have also come a long way from the white cloths used in earlier times. Cloth diapers now come in different clothes laced with baby friendly designs and colors, and also include waterproof bands around the legs and waist to avoid leaks. They are also able to absorb almost as much as disposable waste with their removable linings. Cloth diapers though more often require diaper changes, since they aren't as absorbent as disposable ones, so keep that in mind.

What Type of Diaper Should I Use if My Twins Attends Day Care?

Many day care centers require disposables for convenience and for health reasons. Most of them will not allow for cloth diapers so parents aren't left with much of a choice.

Which Type of Diaper Best Keeps Diaper Rash at Bay?

Cloth diapers tend to be more comfortable and breathable, while they also do a great task as long as you can ensure you get it changed as quick as it soiled. Disposables, allow for your baby to be kept comfortable and dry for longer periods, because of their absorbing creams. The absorbent gels hold huge amount of fluids and can keep them away from your baby's skin. This means your baby's skin is kept dry longer, also minimizing skin contact with urine and even some parts of stool. There are also breathable disposable diapers with material that support air flow to your infants' skin. Also various disposable diaper brands now contain protective coating substances that keep the skin protected, like barrier creams the likes of Balmex do. However some babies develop heat or skin rashes while wearing disposable diapers, it could be an allergic trigger, or the diaper being too tight. If this is the case, experiment with a distinct size or brand, or you can switch to traditional cloth diapers.

Making the Decision.

The right choice depends on what suits your family's needs and lifestyle. Development in production technology has improved the options available for both cloth and disposable diapers. Nothing stops you from using a combination of both, other a parents have actually done the same. For example, some use cloth diapers for newborns and younger babies, while using disposables for toddlers who are more active, or some use disposables during the night, so as not to interrupt sleep on wet diapers and cloth diapers during the day, or you could also decide to use cloth diapers at home and disposables when you're outside or travelling.

Cutting on costs:

As the cost of diapers for twins and multiples can be heavy, here are some tips to help get some savings:

Know how much your diapers cost

The first step to saving is to understand how much the cost is per diaper. This allows you to calculate and decide if a sale is great or not, or if you can couple it with coupons or other discounts for a good deal. This way, no matter what brands you choose, (considering price points or discounts tend to be higher for brands Pampers compared to Luvs), you know what a good deal is for each brand and each size.

Buy in Bulk!

Watch out for discount promos sales for buying bigger packs of diapers. They may not come too often, but you'll find that the cost per diaper tends to be lower (they also often come with a couple of free diaper pieces with larger packs). So the bigger packs or boxes of diapers you buy the better.

Store Branded Diapers and Wipes Are Just as Good as Expensive brands

The expensive brands are known for quality, but you'll find that store brands do just as well if not better. Savvy parents also make savings from mixing them up with branded disposable diapers. They use the cheapest in the daytime at home, and then use the more expensive ones during travel or at night time for sleep time.

Always check for quality, despite the cost. Some diapers may be cheaper but can only hold half as much fluids, so you end up with using more diapers in a pack. In the long run, you end up spending more than you thought you saved. For wipes, generic brands aren't too different from branded ones, they also come in fragrance-free and hypo-allergenic types.

Use Amazon Mom

You can save 20% off of diapers through an Amazon Mom's Membership with their Subscribe & save subscription. In addition to this, you also get $1 to $3 e-coupons regularly. Amazon also offers price matching for Walmart items, as it's their biggest competitor. That and your 20% savings makes a very good deal! Apart from saving on diapers with your membership, you can also enjoy a 15% baby registry discount.

Prevent Wasteful Purchases

Wipes tend to dry out when not used which also means you can't buy them in bulk, unlike with diapers. Soft packed wipes are particularly the ones that dry out easier even when sealed.

So to avoid wasting your budget, buy wipes in plastic containers if you plan to buy in bulk. You can also save the plastic containers and refill them with soft packed wipes. Also make sure to store unopened soft packed whites in a closed space while you aren't using them.

If your stored wipes seem a little dry, you can easily get them moist again with a bit of warm water. It sounds simple and logical, but you'll be surprised at how many parents throw away their boxes of wipes just because they seemed a bit dry!

Chapter 10

Breastfeeding twins

There are several different positions you can use to nurse your twins at the same time. One way is to make their legs overlap while they face in front of you, so they are making an X across your lap. Another good approach is to position your twins in the clutch hold, to help support this position place pillows at your side (and perhaps another on your lap) then place them on the pillows with their legs positioned towards the back of the chair. Keep in mind that when you place your twins in front of you, you have to keep their whole bodies facing toward you, have their chests facing your chest and their bodies shouldn't be facing up. This is very important to ensure your babies get enough milk and that you are kept comfortable, avoiding any soreness.

You can also use a lot of pillows and even buy special nursing pillows made for rearing twins. It is also ideal to alternate feeding each baby from both breasts, as it helps even out their feeding needs.

There are many different positions to breastfeed, and learning them will help you adjust to your surroundings as you feed them, and find which ones both you and your babies will be most comfortable in. Nursing while lying down tends to be quite tricky to learn, particularly on your first few weeks breastfeeding, but learning how to do it will help you get some rest as you nurse.

Always remember to hydrate and feed yourself. Moms tend to forget about caring for themselves when they're too excited and busy with their little ones. When you have to provide breast milk for twins, you'll need to add about 1,000 additional calories to your daily diet. Needless to say, a crash diet is not going to be ideal for you. To provide enough for your babies, you need to follow a sensible, well-balanced breastfeeding diet and keep yourself hydrated with lots of water.

Be ready if one of your babies finishes feeding earlier than the other. If this happens and you are alone, make sure you have some toys on hand ready to keep the one of your babies busy while the other continues to feed. Some babies find breastfeeding relaxing and will just fall asleep, but is best to be prepared so you don't end up scrambling when they happen to be awake.

Sometimes one breast gives less milk less than the other – it's normal so don't worry about that. Some moms seem to produce a good supply from the right; and very little from the left. This is also one reason why alternating your babies between breasts is important. You can also decide to swap them midway of their feeding. You'll also find that your babies will have a different level of force when they suck, so switching them will also allow your body to get used to it on both of your breasts.

Follow a flexible nursing schedule

Simultaneously feeding your babies is the most optimal use of your precious time, and keeping a flexible schedule to feed them is ideal. You'll find though that your twins, no matter how alike, can be different in this particular area, one of them might have a bigger appetite than the other and may want to be fed every 2 hours, while the other would be fine at 3 hour intervals between feedings. Some moms advise that following the hungrier baby's feeding time for both works best for them, while some moms simply nurse on demand during the day, while following a fixed schedule at night.

Signs That All's Well:

Your twins feed at least every 2-3 hours or a total of at least 8 times in a day for their first 2-3 weeks.

With this frequency of feeding, they should also produce at least 3 stools per day, which will lighten in color to yellowy-mustard on the 5th day after their birth.

They should be gaining about an ounce a day in weight come their 5th day after being born and through the remainding first 3 months.

They wet about 7-8 cloth diapers a day or 5-6 disposables. It is hard to tell when disposable diapers are wet since they are more absorbent. So if you aren't sure, you can take it off and compare its weight vs. an unused disposable diaper.

Note: Wet diapers alone are not enough to tell if a baby is dehydrated. Even with the lack of milk they will still wet a diaper. The best ways to check are still looking at the output of their stools and how well they are gaining weight. If they do seem to be peeing less, it doesn't do harm to check other symptoms or check with your baby's pediatrician.

Nursing Wear

You need to feel comfortable while nursing. Stress and discomfort doesn't help with your milk supply. A nursing wardrobe isn't any good without a good nursing bra or tank. You can opt to wear a regular bra that you can flip up or pull aside, but this tends to loosen them and will make you lose support faster. Nursing bras and tanks provide better support and convenience since they have special snaps, clips, or hooks that allow a section of the fabric to fold down without changing the bra's support structure.

Nursing on the Go

Don't be embarrassed to nurse in public! You have the right to do so and every mom who breastfeeds their babies should be very proud of themselves. If you prefer some privacy while you nurse your babies in public, a nursing cover will be very useful. It keeps both you and your babies comfortable since it gives you enough privacy, while hiding your babies from visual distractions as they feed.

Chapter 11

Twin Pregnancy Resources

People with twins have special twin groups which you can join. Twin communities are vastly available. These support groups are made up of parents with twins who share their own experiences which you can learn from. In these groups, you will share each others experiences about carrying and delivering twins, bringing them up as well as advising each other if needed. There is nothing as good as sharing experiences and laughter with other mothers who have already been there!

Here are some of the recommended resources thst parents of twins, triplets and those who are expecting can turn to:

US Government and Non-Profit Assistance

You can get assistance if you are raising twins from the government, non-profit organizations and other resources.

These include and are not limited to:

- Medicaid
- Federal Public House Assistance
- Women Infants and Children WIC

- Car Seat Assistance Program
- Diaper Banks
- Meals for Children Programs such as School Breakfast Program SBP, National School Lunch Program (NSLP) and others.
- Companies' Samples, Discounts and Multiple Programs, and many more.

Babies in Belly

You may want to sign up to an exercise class. Babies in Belly offers you pre-natal exercises which you can do in the comfort of your home.

Multiple Births: Prenatal Education and Bereavement Support

This website is educational and offers prenatal and post-natal information while addressing commonly asked questions and concerns.

Twins List

Twins List helps members share their opinions and comments on various topics. The topics range from those that advise about potty training to school life and much more.

Twins Day Festival

Twins Day Festival is a gathering based in Ohio for day of fun for all twins and multiples whether they are young or old. It involves their parents too. Its a once in a lifetime opportunity to share your joy and experiences with other parents and multiples across the country.

Final Words

Raising twins is very rewarding although it calls for efficiency and dedication. However, it is very convenient in that, some problems you encounter with a singleton, you will only handle them once or simultaneously.

If you are a first time parent it may also be too overwhelming because there is not much time to learn from past mistakes when bringing up twins, but I truly hope the information in this book has helped you overcome many of these hurdles.